THE PRETEEN'S
FIRST BOOK ABOUT
LOVE, SEX, AND AIDS

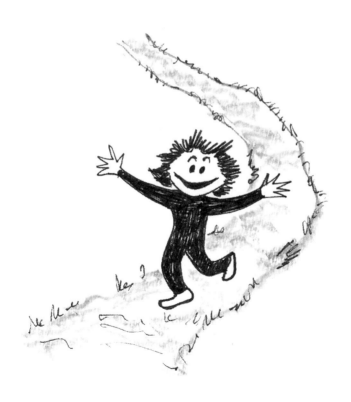

THE PRETEEN'S FIRST BOOK ABOUT LOVE, SEX, AND AIDS

Michelle Harrison, M.D.

Illustrations by
Lynn Beckstrom

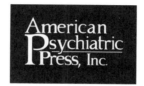

American Psychiatric Press, Inc.

Washington, DC
London, England

Copyright © 1995 Michelle Harrison, M.D.
ALL RIGHTS RESERVED
Manufactured in the United States of America on acid-free paper
98 97 96 95   4 3 2 1
First Edition

American Psychiatric Press, Inc.
1400 K Street, N.W., Washington, DC   20005

Library of Congress Cataloging-in-Publication Data
Harrison, Michelle.
    The preteen's first book about love, sex, and AIDS / Michelle
Harrison ; illustrated by Lynn Beckstrom. — 1st ed.
        p.   cm.
    ISBN 0-88048-698-8
    1. Sex instruction for children.   2. Love—Juvenile literature.
3. Man-woman relationships—Juvenile literature.   4. Hygiene,
Sexual—Juvenile literature.   I. Beckstrom, Lynn.   II. Title.
HQ53.H375   1995   94-34116
                                                            CIP
                                                            AC

British Library Cataloguing in Publication Data
A CIP record is available from the British Library.

CONTENTS

INTRODUCTION: TO THE READER

*I*f you are about to be a teen—or are even already a teen—some important questions are on your mind:

- ✓ WHO WILL LOVE ME?
- ✓ IS LOVE THE SAME AS A CRUSH?
- ✓ WHAT DOES IT MEAN TO BE SEXUAL?
- ✓ IS SEX THE SAME AS LOVE?
- ✓ SHOULD I HAVE SEX?
- ✓ HOW CAN I BE SAFE FROM AIDS?
- ✓ WILL SEX MAKE ME FEEL GROWN-UP?
- ✓ WILL SEX MAKE ME HAPPY?
- ✓ HOW WILL I KNOW?
- ✓ WHO CAN I TRUST?
- ✓ WHO WILL I LOVE?

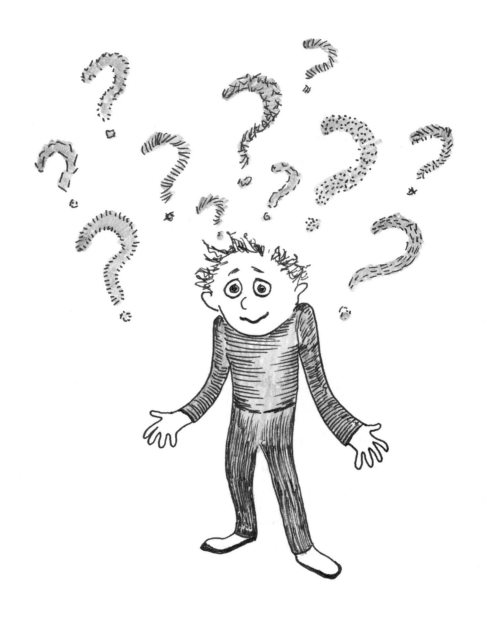

THE PRETEEN'S FIRST BOOK ABOUT LOVE, SEX, AND AIDS

Growing up is sometimes hard to do. Everyone seems to eventually, but each one of us does it a little differently. Some of us grow faster in some ways than others. Our bodies may *seem* grown-up long before our emotions and attitudes grow up. Or we may *feel* grown-up before our bodies really mature. There is no one right speed or pace or pattern for leaving childhood.

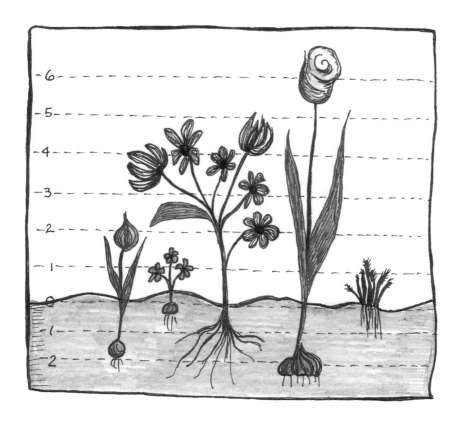

In addition, our families, religions, and cultures have different expectations of how we should think and behave about love, our bodies, and sex. This book is about helping you find *your* answers to your questions about love, sex, and AIDS.

There have always been risks to having sex—risks like pregnancy, sexually transmitted diseases, and hurt feelings. But AIDS has changed the way we all think about love, and especially about sex. Love and sex may be what you *want* to think about, but AIDS is what you end up *having* to think about.

You aren't the only one with these tough questions, and you don't have to search all alone. Others—parents, teachers, doctors, clergy, and friends—may not always have all the answers, or the right answers for you, but they may be able to listen and help you find your way.

Love and sex are not simple matters, not for teens *or for grown-ups*. Sexual feelings can and do occur without love.

❤ *YOU CAN LOVE SOMEONE AND NOT WANT TO HAVE SEX.*

❤ *LOVE IS A FEELING. SEX IS AN ACTIVITY.*

❤ *YOU CAN WANT TO HAVE SEX AND NOT LOVE SOMEONE.*

You experience sexual feelings mostly in relation to other people, so sex is also about your relationships with other people. Sometimes you may think about sex in relation to real people you know. Other times you may have sexual fantasies about people you don't know—like movie stars or singers. So, part of thinking about sex is thinking about someone else.

While sex hasn't changed since your parents were your age, the risks have. Many forms of birth control are available, although surprise pregnancies still happen because people of all ages just don't use them, or don't use them correctly. At the same time, the epidemic of AIDS has created a terrible new fear. What hasn't changed at all are the mixed-up emotions that adults and teens have when thinking about sex. We —your parents, teachers, doctors, friends, and other adults you trust—need to understand how we can help you create paths through the pleasure, fear, and confusion of sexuality.

You can find sex everywhere around you. Whether you are looking at jeans, cars, or eyeglasses, sex is the lure. You've watched TV and movies in which happiness and sex are said to be the same. You've also watched the news and seen violence in schools and streets and between countries. The backdrop of your childhood has been the threat of random danger from strangers, breakfast tables set with milk cartons showing pictures of missing children, and everywhere, crime, drugs, alcohol, drive-by killings, and now AIDS!

Sex has been sold to you as the path to happiness, but it also carries the threat of death from AIDS. It's natural to be curious, eager, and scared all at the same time. In fact, it's hard not to be very confused.

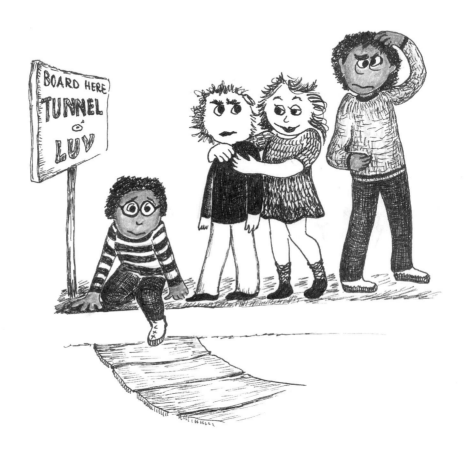

Some of your friends may be thinking a lot about sex. Others may still have months or years to go before they begin to think about it. We all have our own pace and our own timing. There is no time limit. It's not a class with grades. It's just finding your own way. It's not a race.

   THE PRETEEN'S FIRST BOOK ABOUT LOVE, SEX, AND AIDS

These days it is hard to separate sex from the fear of AIDS. What used to worry parents and teens now causes panic. Because you are probably not going to give up thinking about sex, new guidelines, new approaches to the questions of sexuality are desperately needed. AIDS forces us to think more about sexuality, its consequences, and our religious and moral beliefs about it.

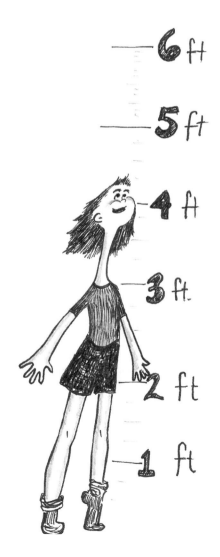

And we adults need to do better than just to try to scare you. We need to give you information and respect your ability to use it to your benefit and for your own safety. We need to trust that you too are struggling with difficult questions that have very complicated answers—answers about trust, love, emotions, sex, and danger.

To do that, first we have to get your attention.

Read on!

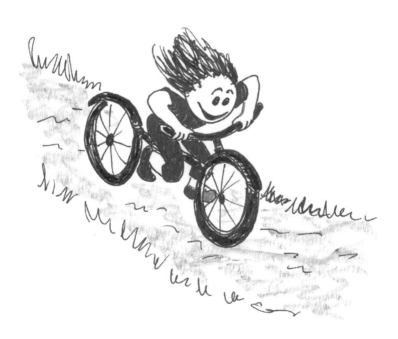

WHY TAKE CARE OF YOUR BODY?

Because doctors tell you to . . . . . . [   ]

Because parents tell you to . . . . . . [   ]

Because teachers tell you to . . . . . [   ]

Because it's the only one you have . . [**X**]

*I*f you, at your age, were suddenly given a car that would be yours for the rest of your life, you would probably set about learning about all of the parts, how to fix it, or at least when to have it fixed or serviced. You would care about its insides as well as its outside. You would know that a paint job doesn't do much good if the engine isn't working right. You would look for the best fuel that

1

you could find and would avoid fuel diluted with water or filled with additives that might clog up the fuel injectors.

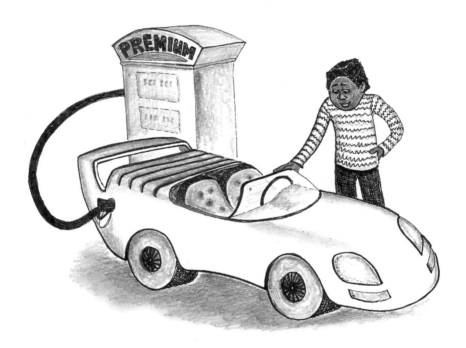

If this were the only car you would ever have, you would have to put up with its defects and try to get the most you could out of it. If you weren't thrilled with it, you might be a little upset; but then, because it was your only car, you'd make the best of it. Well, wouldn't you?

Actually, people never seem totally satisfied with their bodies. Every person—kid or adult—seems to think it would be better to be either taller or shorter, thinner or fatter, lighter or darker. Learning to live with the body you have can be a challenge to everyone, but especially to kids whose bodies do give them major problems. Kids want to feel just like everyone else, so having a body that's different, or difficult, can be a real challenge. You have to remember that a body is only a part of you. Cars don't make us who we are, and neither do bodies. And you also have to remember that everyone feels some sense of being different or of not being good enough.

You—teens, little brothers and sisters, big brothers and sisters, and even parents—sometimes feel like you will live forever and that nothing can hurt you. You just can't imagine anything that would destroy you. Sometimes it's good to feel that self-confident, but sometimes it leads people to take dangerous risks. While adults and religious leaders may argue about the nature of immortality and of the soul, they all agree that being a person, as we experience it, ends when the body is destroyed. Once the car is totaled, the driver is useless.

The human body generally stays healthy unless you do things to harm it. Some of the most harmful things are alcohol, cigarettes, and drugs. Alcohol damages your liver and your brain. Cigarettes leave thick deposits of charcoal in your lungs so as you get older, your lungs will not work as well, and you are more likely to get lung cancer. Drugs destroy all parts of you—brain and body.

Unfortunately, people sometimes think that these substances are cool or will make them feel grown-up. Friends who drink, smoke, or do drugs may want you to try them too. Those people *need* for you to do those things too, so they can convince themselves that they aren't doing anything dangerous, because after all, now *you* are doing it too. You may see the adults around you smoking or drinking, and you may think that if they can do it, so can you. But you really can be smarter than some of the grown-ups around you. You can take better care of your body. It's O.K. to want to live, to want to be safe, to want to have a healthy body.

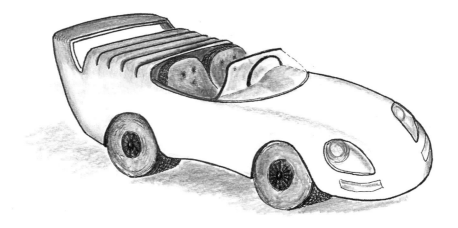

ABOUT LOVE

*T*o *love and be loved.* It's what we all want; it's what we all try for. But how do we know? How do we ever know?

Adults say to teens, "Sex is only for when you love someone." Then the teen says, "How will I know if it's really love?" We usually say, "You'll know."

But knowing if what you feel is love is not so easy. If you made a list of the parts of love, it would look something like this:

❤ *ATTRACTION*

❤ *AFFECTION*

❤ *WANTING TO BE TOGETHER*

❤ *BEING HAPPY WHEN YOU'RE TOGETHER*

❤ *A SENSE OF ONENESS WITH THE OTHER PERSON*

❤ *A SENSE OF SHARED FATE*

❤ *A SENSE OF SPIRITUAL CONNECTION*

5

The trouble is . . . all these features of love can be there without real or lasting love being present. In other words, none of those feelings happen only when we are in love. It is possible to feel and believe all the experiences and sensations listed here—to feel some or all of them *deeply*—and yet to have them change quickly. Attraction can become disgust; wanting to be with someone can become a wish never to see the person again. What seemed to be someone's best qualities can become what you most dislike. A sense of shared fate can evaporate into a feeling that the relationship is meaningless.

Obsession can also look like love. The term "fatal attraction," from the title of a movie, is often used to describe an obsession that makes you believe your survival depends on being with a particular person. You may want to totally control the other person or feel yourself controlled by him or her. You may feel lost, as though you do not really exist apart from that person.

Love between two people can only exist as long as you both exist separately and independently. But, not to scare you—lots of people (adults and teens alike) *fantasize* or *daydream* that they can't live without the person they love.

Love is an experience of feeling and behavior over time. At any one moment, all you can say is that you feel love right now. In other words, attraction, sexual desire, and love may all start out looking and feeling the same. There is no test of love except the passage of time.

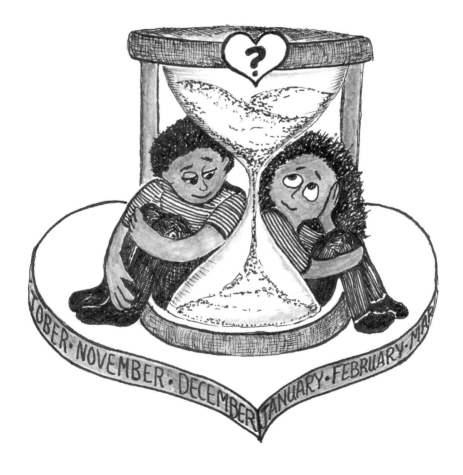

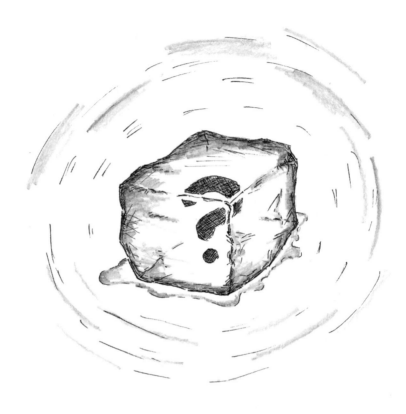

On the surface it might not seem that ice cubes and diamonds could help us to understand love. But maybe they can.

Picture a diamond buried deep inside an ice cube. From the surface of the ice cube, you cannot see the diamond, because it is too similar to the ice crystals. On the surface, an ice cube with a diamond looks like all other ice cubes. It is only with the passage of time—the melting of the ice—that you can see whether or not a diamond is hidden inside. In the beginning, most relationships may seem to be the same and seem to hold the same powerful emotions. When you "fall in love," you can't tell whether this is love. You just won't know for a while. The problem of whether what you feel is enduring or fleeting is not unique to you. It is equally difficult for people who are 13, 18, 30, 40, or 60. When you are "in love," you just have to live with your feelings and wait to see what happens as the ice cube melts. Is it a cube with a diamond, or does it all become a puddle of water?

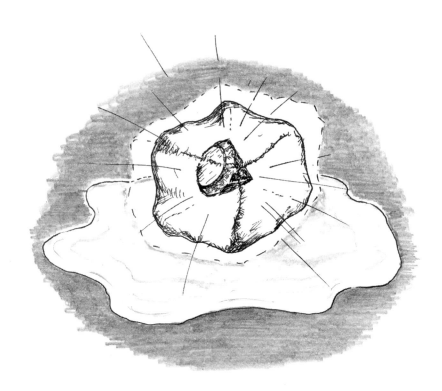

Well, what are you to do while you wait for the ice cube to melt? Actually, there are ways to get hints about whether or not what you have with this person is love and whether the feelings will stand the test of time.

- Are you friends? In other words, can you really say how you feel?
- Can you spend happy, nonromantic time together—time working or studying or playing together?
- Can you confide in this person? Can you trust his or her confidentiality? Can he or she keep a secret?
- What are the things you agree and disagree about? Can you talk about it if you disagree over music, politics, religion, or ideals? The issue is not whether you agree, but how you deal with differences. Can you disagree without angry outbursts, or sulky silences, or intimidation, or competition?
- Are you free to say no? This is important for both boys and girls. None of you should feel forced to do anything that feels uncomfortable. It's not love when someone makes you feel unsafe or used.

How does this person treat other friends? How have previous romances ended? Has this person been mean or spiteful, or are old boyfriends or girlfriends treated with respect?

None of the answers to these questions can tell you whether you love someone, or if you are loved. But if there are problems with any of these questions, it's time to be cautious and to take a "wait and see" attitude. Sometimes the relationship has already become more physical than one of you wants, but there's no reason you can't back off for a while and give the ice cube time to melt.

Love means trusting and respecting your own need for safety—and your friend's need for it, too.

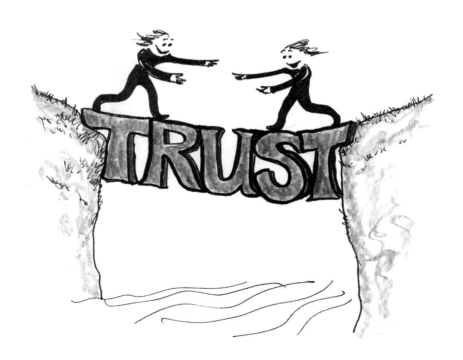

SEX

BRAIN, BODY, AND BEHAVIOR

Sex is about what you feel (physically and emotionally), what you think, and then what you do—or don't do. While feelings often come from the body, decisions about what to do about the feelings are made in the head—even when it doesn't seem that way. When it *seems* as though we are just giving in to our feelings, in fact we are making a decision to let our feelings determine what we do. We are making a decision not to interfere with what our feelings and bodies seem to be telling us to do.

People don't usually think about the brain when they are learning or thinking about sexuality. But the brain is the communications and decision center. It's the place that takes in all the information and feelings from inside the body; it considers the advice of parents, teachers, and friends; it rummages through its own memories and values. Then it makes final decisions on how to act or not act. Sexual feelings may be located in the body, but it's the brain that decides what to do, or not do. *That's* not always so easy!

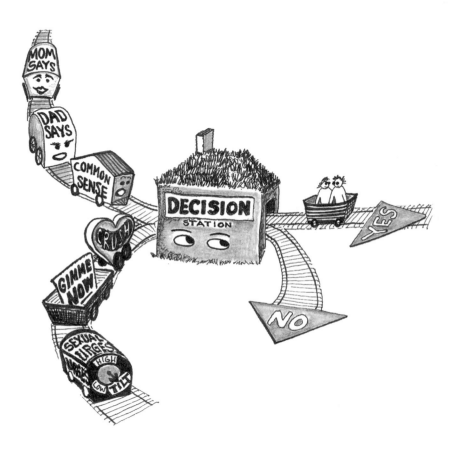

Thinking about your body sexually is different from thinking about it physically or athletically. When you are playing sports, what matters most is how your body works—how strong it is, how fast you can run, how far you can hit a ball. But sex isn't about accomplishments or performance—even though some people think it is. It's about how you think your body *looks* and *feels*, what and who you are thinking about, and who you are with. People actually *think* about sex more than they ever behave sexually. Sometimes sexual feelings can feel like they are stronger than your brain. Physical feelings can be overpowering at times.

Just think about what goes on in the brain about sexuality. First of all, it's where thoughts are, where images and daydreams are; it's where memories are. When you hear or see or write the word *sex*, your brain automatically makes an image, or many images, and sets off a series of memories, thoughts, and pictures, all of which are happening in your brain. When you have sexual feelings, they appear as images and emotions. You imagine all sorts of situations. You may imagine kissing, or touching, or just looking at someone. You may even be much happier just daydreaming rather than doing anything sexual.

SIGNALS FROM YOUR BODY

The body has centers that seem to collect and generate sexual feelings. Nerves (which are like telephone lines) from all parts of the body communicate sensations to the brain. Years ago in school, you learned about the body's senses: sight, sound, smell, taste, touch, and the ability to know where your arms and legs are (the kinesthetic sense). Those senses are, at various times, involved in sexual feelings and sensations. You see, it's not just the sensation or ability to feel that makes a feeling sexual. It's the setting, who you are with, and how you are feeling in general.

Let's use kissing, for example. Thinking about kissing can take a lot of time. The hours or minutes or seconds you spend actually kissing aren't that many. But daydreaming about it, having mixed feelings about it, and then reliving it can take up a lot of time in your life.

What is kissing anyway, and why do you want it? As with any physical experience, kissing when you don't want to is terrible. Putting your lips on someone else's can seem disgusting, unless of course you like that person, and then whatever they do may seem to feel good. But just think about it. It's not the kiss itself that turns you on. Do you look forward to sloppy kisses on the lips from grandparents, aunts and uncles, Labrador retrievers, or babies?

Kissing is special because when it feels warm or close, and it is with someone you *want* to be touching you, it gives you a good feeling; it gives you good thoughts. You kiss with your mouth, but the feelings from your mouth have meaning when mixed with your thoughts and emotions.

We often talk about *sexual development*, and what we mean is that some parts of the body change, but

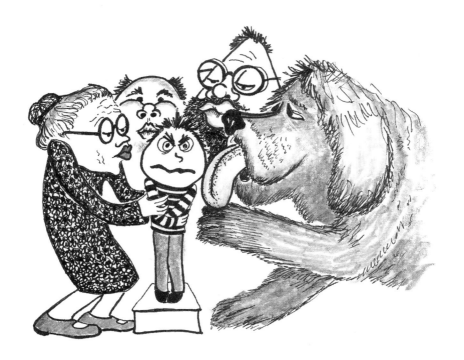

also that they take on a different meaning. They represent, or symbolize, sexuality. However, you may not experience your body changes in that way, and you may not respond to someone else's sexual development in that way. You may find that some thoughts or pictures give you sensations in different parts of your body. That may be pleasant, or it may be scary, or both. No part of sex is separate from the rest of your life, how you feel, or what you think.

For girls, breast development symbolizes an increase in sexual development. Your breast development often leaves *other* people thinking that having breasts is the same as feeling sexual. Breast development may signal to other people that a girl is becoming a woman, or is more "mature" or "ready," but it says nothing about how the girl actually feels. Big breasts may make other people, like boys or parents, think that a girl is *more* sexual than she feels, when she may still feel like a little kid with foreign breasts stuck onto her.

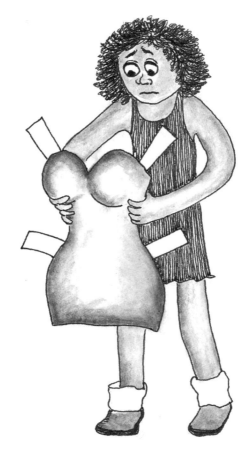

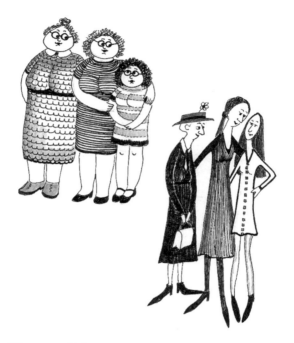

Girls with small breasts may be considered uninterested in sex when they might actually be very interested. They may be ignored by boys because the boys may think that small breasts mean that a girl isn't interested in boys. Breast development is part of the way a girl's body matures, but it says nothing about her feelings or interest in sexuality or her emotional maturity—or anything else, for that matter.

Most of a girl's breast size is related to heredity, as well as to her weight. When girls put on weight, their breasts sometimes become bigger too. You get your breast size from your families, for the most part, not from your interest in sex.

Some boys may have slight breast enlargement, especially if they are husky. Deposits of fatty tissue in the breast may be an embarrassment to boys. Enlarged breasts don't make a boy any less male. Remember the brain—that's what's important. It's how you feel about sexuality, what kind of daydreams or fantasies you have, what you decide to do or not to do, that describes your sexuality, not what you look like to others. That's true whether you are a boy or a girl.

The greatest area of sexual concentration is the genitals. It's the part of our bodies that is most covered up in our culture, and in fact in almost all cultures. Even in places where men, and sometimes women, go bare above the waist, an uncovered genital area is extremely unusual. Generally, as humans, what we think about most is what we cover up the most—maybe with the hope that if it can't be seen, it isn't there.

For the growing young man, what's hiding there? Well, the little boy is becoming a big boy.

You boys have been wondering all those years how your little penises would *ever* get to be as big as your father's or uncle's or big brother's. . . . Well, for some of you that wondering has come to an end, and for some there is still some time to go. Your genitals grow at different rates. Some of you have new hairy places, and growing parts that sometimes seem to act without your will. Boys' penises may become hard and stick out at the most embarrassing times—in class, at the beach, at home with family.

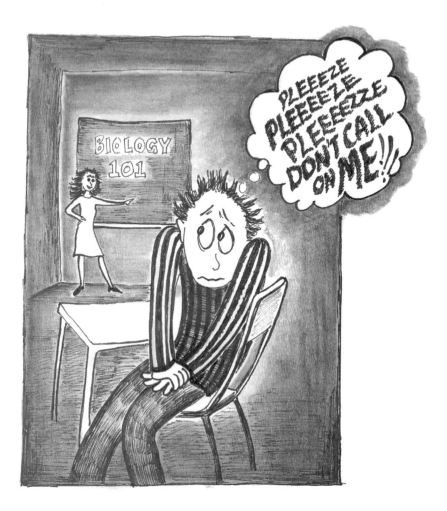

Boys often have "wet dreams" in which they may dream about sex and wake up with erections. Or they may have dreams and ejaculate—when sexual arousal leads to semen coming out of the penis.

And for those boys who so far haven't been covering themselves up around the house, suddenly the cover goes on.

School bathrooms become a place where boys learn not to notice the size of the kid peeing in the next urinal, all the while desperately wondering how you really compare. This can be a difficult time for boys. In some ways, worrying about their penis size may become the symbol of their worth, or how "manly" or how strong they are. But, like breast size for girls, penis size also has more to do with heredity and other biological factors than "how much of a man" you are or ever will be.

Girls have a more complicated relationship to their genital area than boys do. It's complicated because mostly there isn't anything to see, and because they may have been given a very wide range of stories about "what little girls have." At some time in the life of every little girl, she notices some unmistakable differences between what she has and what little boys have.

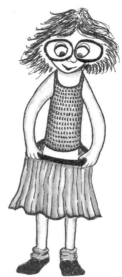

She may have discovered the difference because she has brothers, or because she saw a baby boy's diaper being changed, or because her mother showed her pictures, or because she saw her father naked. She may have been told, "But your parts are inside," leaving her to imagine hidden genitals. Or she may have been told, "But you have a wonderful vagina!" which may also have left her puzzled. She may have done some exploring on her own. And she may have decided to just not think about it anymore when told that a baby might pass though an opening there one day.

Girls become familiar with their genitals when they begin to menstruate—when they get their periods—and then it's impossible to ignore the changes in their bodies. Suddenly, although you may still feel like a little kid, you have to worry about sanitary pads or tampons, and whether you can swim, and how to make sure no one notices you are bleeding. If you have cramps too, you may be very unhappy about the changes in your body. Cramps are no fun, and they can seem to spoil the idea of that "wonderful vagina."

Girls may begin to have sexual feelings radiating from their vaginal area. There is a tiny area, called the clitoris, at the top of the vaginal area, just inside the labia (or lips) of the genital area, that is similar in some ways to the male penis. Girls may have very intense sexual feelings when the clitoris is touched. The feelings may be pleasant, or they may be frightening and distracting. Again, it depends on the setting, what the girl is thinking about, and how she feels about sexual feelings, herself, and her body.

BODIES THAT ARE CHALLENGED

Kids with disabilities—whether they have trouble walking, seeing, hearing, speaking, or even thinking—wonder about love as much as everyone else. You may have a disability that is obvious, like being in a wheelchair, or less obvious, like trouble with your eyesight. But whether or not your disability is obvious to others, you probably think of yourself as different, and others may too.

When it comes to movies, TV, and talk about love and sexuality, you may feel left out. Remember, Hollywood really is make-believe, and few kids really look or feel like the ones you see. So, if you have a disability, you aren't alone in wishing you were like the stars.

But there are special problems for kids with disabilities. You may not be able to be as independent as other kids, and the adults around you might get used to having to do a lot for you. You will probably be treated like a child longer than others. For all kids, it's hard to separate when parents are just being normally protective from when they are overprotective. But it's even harder when parents have had to do more for you because of your disability.

Whatever the condition of your body, whatever your disabilities or challenges, your feelings and dreams are just the same as the rest of the gang's. You worry about who you will love and who will love you. What is different sometimes is figuring out how to have a fun social life, and what particular problems you will confront because of your body. This is a time to talk to older kids and adults in similar circumstances. This is a time to have honest talks with the adults around you about what you want. And this is also a time *not* to assume that you will be rejected because of your disabilities. There are a lot of kids out there who will think of you as a person, and just accept your disability . . . and a lot of kids out there who also feel different, even if they don't look it.

We all have to struggle with the same problems of love, intimacy, sexuality, trust, and AIDS—no matter who we are. In that respect, we are all challenged.

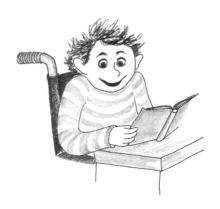

WHAT YOUR PARENTS WORRY ABOUT

Sex . . . . [X]
Pregnancy . . . . [X]
AIDS . . . . [X]

SEX

You would think that as people get older they would understand sex more. Well, that doesn't seem to happen. What they usually know is more of the "how to," but they remain as confused as ever about what it all means. So, they figure if *they* still don't understand it, how can you be expected to know what it is all about and to be responsible about sexual behavior?

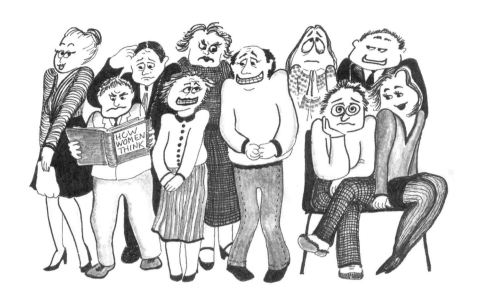

Sex is very hard to be responsible about. It's not always a part of our lives that is well thought out. Sometimes it seems that sexual feelings make decisions for us, instead of our making decisions about sexual feelings. It is hard to be in control of what you don't understand. It's hard to be in control when your thinking and feelings are opposite to each other. It's also hard when others around you may be saying, "But everyone else is doing it!"

And there are usually not many people with whom you can talk about your feelings or questions or uncertainties. Grown-ups get confused too. They may have "affairs" in part because their sexual feelings are strong enough to affect major decisions in their lives. Some may leave marriages and children because someone else comes along. But teens are supposed to have self-control, sometimes more than some of their parents seem to have.

Sometimes grown-ups are worried about teens and sex because their own experiences may not have been so good. The grown-ups' secret is that for many adults, sex isn't—and sometimes never was—a very good experience. TV and movies suggest that everyone goes to bed and has a good time, but the truth is very different. So, part of trying to keep you from having sex before you are older is trying to keep you from the bad times as well as the good.

PREGNANCY

Your parents would probably prefer that you not become a parent until you are ready to be a mom or dad—and *they* are ready to be grandparents. If you as a teenage girl become a mother, or you as a teenage boy become a father, your parents would suddenly be grandparents—without their ever doing anything. That thought can be very frightening to some parents. If you were to become a parent, they might also feel guilty, believing that they must have done something wrong in raising you (or that others will think that they did). They worry about whether you will get to do all the things you want to do in your life if you become a parent too early.

Some parents are scared about unplanned pregnancies because their own track record on birth control may not be so good. In fact, many of you reading this book may have come into this world as a result of an unplanned pregnancy. That is true of most pregnancies throughout the world. Every time adults think about what *they* were like, they get more scared about what you may do.

You see, as a species, we humans might not reproduce if we had to think about it in advance. The possibility of pregnancy is like the default drive on a computer. The basic programming for when males and females have sex is for reproduction. It's automatic—unless it's prevented. That, however, doesn't mean that *you* have to have a baby every time you have sex. Unlike computers, we people can (hopefully) think about what we are doing and try to bring about the results we want. *A lot of learning about sex is learning to separate what we want from what we really must have.*

What if having babies had been linked to food? What if every time you went to the local ice cream shop with your friends and had a hot fudge sundae, you might get pregnant? You'd have to stop and think about how much you wanted the sundae, or you'd have to think about what you could do to prevent becoming a parent if you really wanted that sundae. And, if you were a boy, you'd think about whether wanting a sundae was worth making this girl you liked into a mother and you into a father. And if you were a girl, you'd think about whether a hot fudge sundae was worth becoming a teenage mother.

Because we make it so hard for you to talk about your questions and confusions about sex, you sometimes end up acting without ever really thinking about what you are doing. And because sexual drive can be so strong (and much harder to resist than a hot fudge sundae), babies can be created, with no such intent on anyone's mind. After all, if there were to be lots of babies, then creating them had to be tied to the strongest (and most confusing) drives we have.

The trouble with birth control is that there isn't any method that is easy, safe, and absolutely certain . . . except, of course, "abstinence" (not doing it at all). *All methods of birth control, in one way or another, require that you acknowledge to yourself that you have made a decision that you are willing to have sexual intercourse.* It's hard to say you "accidentally" have a condom or diaphragm in your wallet or purse.

And, for females, many of the methods available to you, such as birth control pills or a diaphragm, require considerable advance planning (like a visit to a doctor or clinic)—and some money. For boys, the practical options for birth control are simpler—like condoms—but still require that you think in advance about what you are doing, how to do it, and how to be prepared.

In the best of all possible worlds, both boys and

girls—and men and women—would think about birth control if they were going to have sex. But unfortunately, in the real world, responsibility for birth control is usually left to the female.

It is quite amazing how people can pretend either that they aren't having sex or that they won't get pregnant. This brings to mind a story . . .

There once was a little boy named David. When David was four, he put a blanket over his face and said to his mommy, "Now you can't see me." He figured that if he couldn't see her, she couldn't see him. In other words, *sometimes we pretend that what can't be seen doesn't exist.*

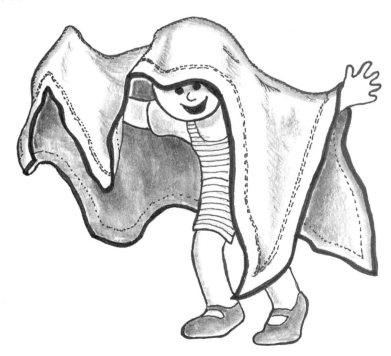

THE PRETEEN'S FIRST BOOK ABOUT LOVE, SEX, AND AIDS

When David was 16, he was going out with Susan. She said she was afraid of getting pregnant. He told her he'd be "careful," and she thought that was enough. He put the bag over his head instead of "you know where," and she got pregnant. Some people will always be four years old.

If you are having trouble with the idea of birth control, just think about *babies.* Don't imagine a cute little bundle of love in your arms. That's hard to resist; and anyway, that's not what raising a baby is like. Instead, imagine a two-year-old puking all night—on you, on the sheets, on towels—running a temperature, and you being scared and wondering what you're doing being a parent at 17 or even younger.

It's not that babies can't be wonderful, and it's not that being a parent isn't also wonderful. But having to raise a child when you are barely out of childhood yourself is very different from daydreams about cute little babies.

A SPECIAL MESSAGE FOR BOYS

Actually, if you are a teenage boy and are reading this book, you are probably trying to be responsible about sexuality. While it is a basic necessity for girls to worry about birth control if they have sex, more and more boys want to share that responsibility. The old images of the macho male didn't allow you boys to have feelings or to be sensitive to the needs of females. And again, AIDS has really forced boys and girls to consider more carefully whether to be sexual with each other.

Pregnancy in teens happens by "accident" when sex may be unplanned and birth control ignored. Or, boys, like girls, may think it would be nice to have a baby. Sometimes boys think of becoming a father as a sign of manhood or being grown-up. They think other people will look up to them. But getting a girl pregnant isn't a symbol of being a man. It's about not controlling where your sperm are, and having one of them go on to make a baby. Sperm make babies, and so if you don't take precautions, your sperm will go on to make babies as often as they are given the chance.

A SPECIAL MESSAGE FOR GIRLS

Having a baby isn't about being a woman. It's about being a teenage mother. Teens become pregnant in the same way adult women become pregnant, but being a teenage mother is much more difficult. As I've said before, getting pregnant is easy if you are having sex. It's not really much of an accomplishment. It just takes one of your eggs and one tiny sperm—and poof! there's a baby inside you.

The major reason for pregnancy (as I said before) is having sex without birth control, which is often the result of having sex without thinking about it in advance. Or you may believe that you are "safe" and just can't get pregnant. Or you may be unhappy in general and think that having a baby to love, and to love you, would make you happy. Or you may think that if you get pregnant, the baby's father will stay with you, that the baby will keep you together. You may see having a baby as a way of getting out of your parents' house, or away from their control. Or you may just be afraid of the uncertainty of what you are doing in your life, and "let" yourself get pregnant as a solution to the question of what to do with your life.

Having a baby may be a wonderful thing to daydream about, but the reality can be a nightmare. Having a baby, whether you are 15 or 30, is a major enterprise. Trying to do it without support—when you haven't figured out yet who you are, who you will love, and what you want to do with your life—is a tough way to spend your teenage years.

You see, doing things with your body, like having sex or making babies—or drinking and smoking—doesn't change who you are or how old you are. Wearing out your body isn't the same as growing up.

AIDS

People who don't want to die are usually afraid of fatal illness. It's natural. They are afraid for themselves, and they are afraid for the people they love. Your parents grew up at a time when it seemed that science had found the cures to more and more illnesses. Smallpox was almost totally wiped out. You've been vaccinated against polio, the epidemic of your parents' childhood. Aside from the tragedy of AIDS itself, it has been a shock to find that a new illness, a new virus, is out of our control. It is made worse because the illness is often tied to sexuality. And anything tied to sexuality reminds people of sex, bodies, goodness, badness, guilt, sin, punishment. . . . Take something we don't understand anyway, tie it to a fatal illness, and you have a lot of scared people. You will learn a lot more about AIDS in the chapter "Sex and AIDS" beginning on page 79.

Parents worry about children. They worry because they love you (you may have mixed feelings about this) and because by the time you reach adolescence, worrying about you has become a habit. They also worry because often they want their children to have, or to be, whatever they have not managed to achieve for themselves. Sometimes that worry feels like a terrible burden to children.

Sometimes children react by being especially cautious, or sometimes by being reckless. Neither response works very well. You have to make sure that you consider your own feelings and dreams, and not only just react to those of other people.

You may be tempted to show your defiance by taking chances about AIDS, but can you take the risk of getting AIDS? The most important thing to remember about AIDS is that you get it from another person. The AIDS virus doesn't live in the air or on trees or in stores. It lives in the body fluids of *other people.* Therefore, the best way to protect yourself is abstinence. The next best way is to know who you are with, and take the proper precautions. You can get AIDS even if you are in love.

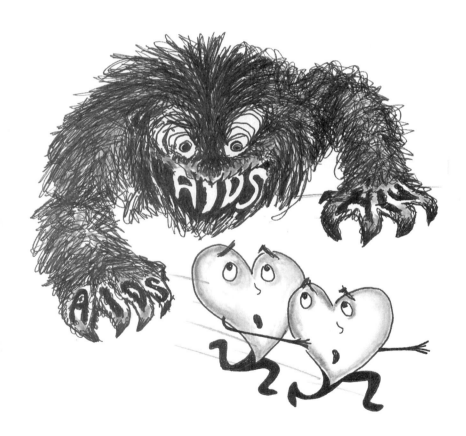

You may be scared to talk about AIDS with someone else your age, but just remember that deep down, all of you are scared. And the only way to bridge that fear is to talk honestly with each other. The other kid is just as scared as you are. If you are really thinking about having sex, then it's essential that you know all about AIDS and how to protect yourself. For that information, see the chapter on "Sex and AIDS" on page 79.

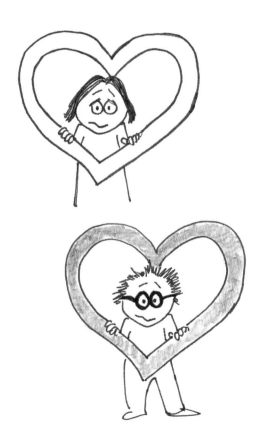

THE STAGES OF
TEEN SEX

BEFORE YOU EVEN START,
GHOSTS
FROM THE PAST

For many of you, going out with another teen or becoming interested or aware of sexual feelings is not your first experience with sex. For some of you this experience was just "child's play" at various stages of childhood. You may have played "doctor" with other children, compared body parts, and played other secret games. All of these are common and usually harmless experiences that children often have with each other. Unfortunately, however, some of us—both boys and girls—may have had frightening, unwanted, and painful sexual encounters, sometimes even with members of our own families, or other people we trusted and looked up to.

Sometimes these experiences happened a long time ago and they are barely remembered. But when you begin to think about love, dating, touching, and sex, the memories may return, and they may even be more vivid and frightening than before. No one should *ever* do anything sexual to you or touch your body or make sexual talk to you *without your permission!* Rape (when someone makes you have some sort of sexual experience by force or threats) and incest (when someone in you family uses power, force, or intimidation to have a sexual encounter with you) are terrible experiences that take a long time to get over—sometimes forever. It makes no difference whether you were molested by a family friend, a teacher, a coach, an older kid, or a stranger in the park. You *always* have the right to say no. *It is **never** your fault if the other person refuses to stop.* These experiences certainly affect your sexual feelings later on. Both boys and girls who have been raped or molested tend to feel shame and guilt. Kids tend to blame themselves for almost everything, even if it's not their fault.

When girls or boys feel bad about themselves, it will affect how they expect others to feel about them. They may seek out people who treat them as badly as they feel about themselves. All these feelings do not go away by themselves, and this is a time to find some help in talking about how you are feeling. If you find yourself with another teen who has been hurt in this way, it is a time for you to be very sensitive and to help him or her find a trusted adult to talk with. Likewise, if it's you who hurts, you need to find someone to talk to. It may be hard to even think about talking to someone about your feelings, but sometimes you can find a special teacher or counselor, or a friend's big sister or brother or parent, or even your own parents.

And this is especially important: don't push yourself or anyone else into any sexual experience that may be frightening for either of you. It's not a cure for the past. This is a time for tenderness and understanding.

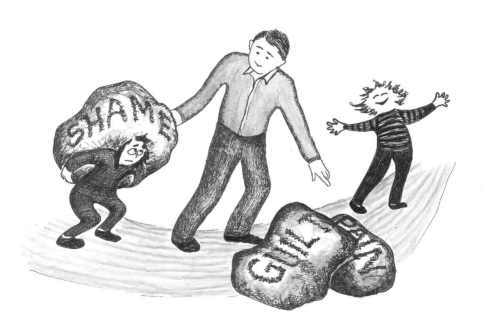

GAMES IN THE DARK... KISSING GAMES

Remember David, with the bag over his head? Well, here he is again, along with Susan and all their friends. They are playing games in the dark. They are pretending that no one can see them—because it's dark. Each one is thinking, "If I don't really see who I'm kissing then I don't have to be responsible for kissing him or her." You shut your eyes, even though the lights are out. It's just another protection against seeing what you are doing. This type of game in the dark is usually played by preteens and younger teens.

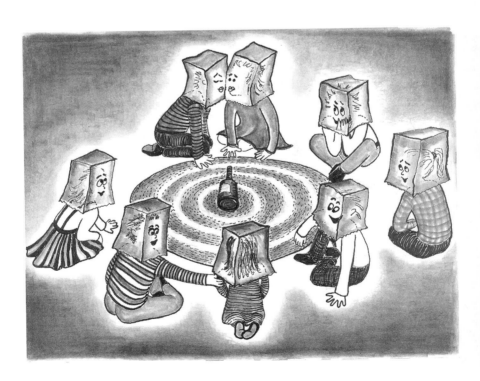

THE PRETEEN'S FIRST BOOK ABOUT LOVE, SEX, AND AIDS

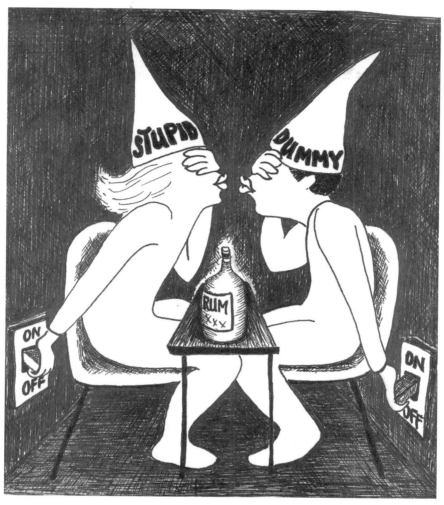

Actually, grown-ups are even better than preteens or teens at playing "games in the dark." Having lived longer and become craftier, and having more independence, adults tend to believe (and maybe it's true) that they can get away with more. Often alcohol is the substitute for the darkness, so they can say, "Well, I was drunk so I didn't know what I was doing."

But like the teen who turns out the light so the games won't be seen, the alcoholic takes the drink that begins to switch off the light of awareness, guilt, and responsibility. Recently, it has become clear that many teens indulge in alcohol- or drug-related "games in the dark." More and more teens, like adults, are drinking so they can act in ways for which they would not want to feel fully responsible.

There is much debate about whether the abuse (or overuse) of alcohol is a sickness or just bad behavior. Whatever the answer, though, alcohol gets a lot of people into a lot of trouble. Alcohol seems to pull the stops on some behaviors. Boys may become more aggressive, both physically and sexually. Girls may become more vulnerable to their feelings and may agree to sexual behavior they would avoid if they weren't drinking. Boys and girls alike may have surges of sadness or anger and may lose control of their feelings and their actions.

GOING OUT

The major accomplishment of adolescence will be to establish whether you can "make the grade." "Going out" (what used to be called dating) is often the test. Like an eight-year-old's playing house or playing Little League, you are practicing for the big time.

Sometimes it feels that if you don't date early, you

won't ever date or won't ever "find a mate." But for those who begin to date late, a fast catching up often occurs. In any event, you really can't date by a textbook schedule, because people grow up differently.

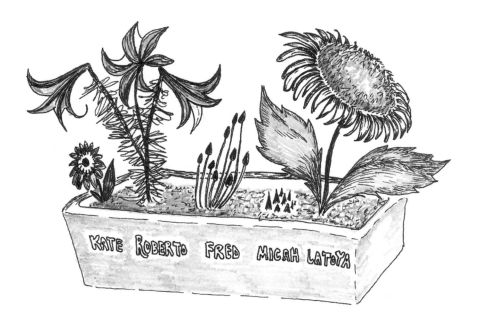

You can have your first date at 19, marry a year later, and have a lifetime marriage. Or, you can date at 14 and still not have found a mate by 30. There just aren't any formulas, no matter what books and movies seem to say.

Adults (parents especially) display a wide and amusing array of attitudes toward teen dating. Some parents are very strict and don't want their teens (especially daughters!) to date until very late.

Parents worry about your ability to use self-control and judgment. Often they remember their own adolescence and some of their confusion about it, and they don't want you to live through everything they did. They don't want you to do all the reckless things they may have done to terrify their own parents—your grandparents.

Other parents may even push their teens to date before they are ready. They worry about your popularity as though it were their own. They get as anxious, or more anxious, than you do about dating and popularity. They get mixed up as to who is the adolescent and relive their own teen years through yours.

Yet other parents, just like little David, put bags over their heads because they can't cope with their child's adolescence, and pretend that nothing is going on.

BODY CONTACT

The problem of becoming too big to sit on a parent's lap is not to be underestimated. While you might not want to be caught dead kissing or hugging a parent, you probably also miss that contact. Being close to another person—touching, hugging, cuddling—is an essential and necessary part of our lives at all ages. Teenagers sometimes crave a lot of hugging. The importance of body contact should never be overlooked. Boys get more body contact than girls through sports and roughhousing. Football, for instance, wouldn't be much without a lot of bodies piled up together. "Well," you might say, "but that's just how the game is played." But *someone* thought up the game, and that someone thought that body contact would be a good idea. And a lot of other people obviously agreed, because it's a popular game.

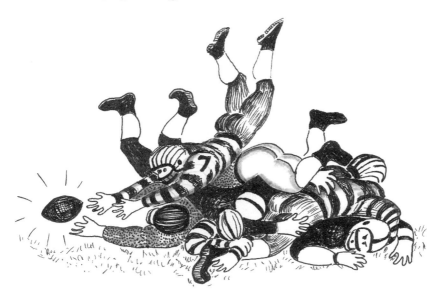

Maybe because boys get more contact in sports, and maybe because they tend to be shy at the thought of touching, all touching that's not related to sports for boys gets lumped into *sex.* Many girls just want cuddling and holding. Sex, or making out, is often just the price they pay for getting the cuddling or touching they want. You boys may be embarrassed at the thought of just wanting close touching, or cuddling. So sometimes you feel you have to look for sex because that's more acceptable than wanting a big hug instead. You worry about what your friends would say if they thought all you wanted was just to be close to someone else.

GOING ALL THE WAY

To score . . . doing it . . . going all the way . . .

Sexual intercourse is when his penis goes into her vagina.

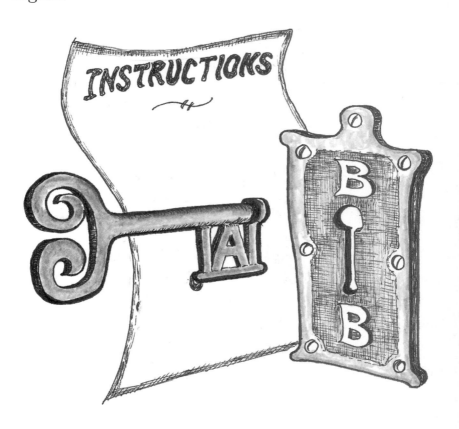

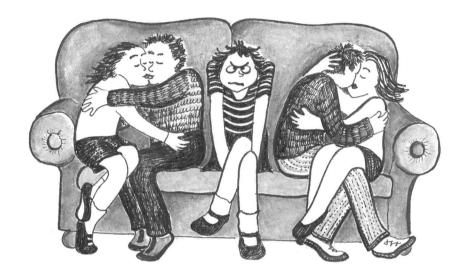

You all learned that years ago. You may have learned it from seeing videos of animals in the wild, or you may have seen two sparrows sitting on a wire together, and then suddenly one pounces on the other. Or you may have had pets—dogs or cats who mated. Most little kids find the whole thing a little disgusting. Somewhere you were also probably told that it wouldn't seem like such a bad idea when you got older. Well, now you are a bit older, but maybe you're still not sure about whether it's disgusting or not. You're withholding final judgment. Maybe you're still convinced it's disgusting and you wouldn't be caught dead doing it, but for the sake of belonging, you're staying quiet on the subject.

Somewhere along the way you've heard some of the following:

- ✓ *"YOU ONLY DO IT FOR LOVE."*
- ✓ *"YOU ONLY DO IT TO HAVE BABIES."*
- ✓ *"YOU ONLY DO IT IF YOU ARE MARRIED."*
- ✓ *"IT GIVES YOU DISEASES."*
- ✓ *"YOU'LL FEEL MORE GROWN-UP IF YOU DO IT."*
- ✓ *"YOU'LL FEEL DIRTY IF YOU DO IT."*
- ✓ *"IT HURTS."*
- ✓ *"IT'S NO BIG DEAL."*
- ✓ *"IT'S THE BEST EXPERIENCE OF YOUR LIFE."*

What is true? People have sexual intercourse for many, many reasons, only some of which are related to sex.

FOR SEXUAL FEELING

This may seem like the most obvious reason for having sex, but it may not be the most common. Eating when you are hungry relieves your hunger. Because having sexual intercourse with another person is so complicated, though, it's not the kind of thing you do just because you feel like it. It's too easy to hurt the other person's feelings, or to feel hurt yourself.

But, believe it or not, sexual intercourse doesn't always satisfy sexual feelings.

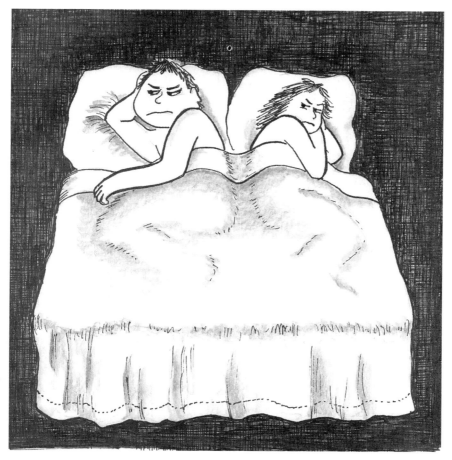

There is a certain amount of learning that takes place, as well as an increasing comfort with your own body. Sometimes when two people have sex, only one of them really enjoys it or feels satisfied. It takes time to learn what kinds of touching or what circumstances give you and your partner pleasure. And it takes a long time to feel able to tell your partner what you like. Practicing at sex is really practicing at talking, communicating, sharing, and loving.

FOR INTIMACY

This is what sex is supposed to be about, in terms of a relationship. Being intimate means being close, or deeply connected, sharing, truly being *with* another person. Ideally, when a girl and a boy or a man and a woman feel close, sex can be—but doesn't have to be— a way of expressing that closeness. Sex with a stranger is not part of closeness, so it's not the sexual activity itself that makes the experience an intimate one. Remember "kissing" and the sloppy kisses from the Labrador retriever? It's not the kiss, but who you are with.

Sex, even with someone you love, if you are not feeling close at that moment is not intimate. Even more important, you can be intimate without being sexual. Sometimes *talking* can be more intimate than having sex, which is why sometimes people find it easier to have sex than to talk seriously or honestly. In talking, you may open up emotional parts of yourself, and that can be very scary.

Sometimes people will take off their clothes and be naked with each other, but they don't feel safe enough to say what they are thinking or feeling. They find it easier to bare their bodies than to bare their emotions.

FOR ATTRACTION

Attraction is what you feel when you get a crush on someone. Suddenly you're "in love," but you don't even know that person or why you are attracted to him or her. That's the ultimate of what parents fear will happen to you . . . because it happens to adults, and it happened to them as teenagers too.

Sometimes adults make stupid choices on the basis of attraction or sex appeal, and they don't want you to be as stupid as they were. Attraction is a great reason to get to know someone better, but having sex may make that more difficult. Sometimes when you get too close too fast, you get scared and feel like you have to run away from the other person altogether.

So, it's not just a matter of "right and wrong" to say that you should take your time to know each other before taking off your clothes. It just works better that way.

FOR FEELING GROWN-UP

When you put on your mother's or your father's clothes, do you really feel grown-up inside?

Well, having sex to feel grown-up doesn't really change how you feel inside. For boys, it may seem like a passage into manhood. For girls, though, it's much more complicated. You may sound grown-up to your friends, but actually, genital activity has never been a good measure of maturity. Too many girls do it to feel grown-up, but they are left feeling more confused and sometimes even younger than before.

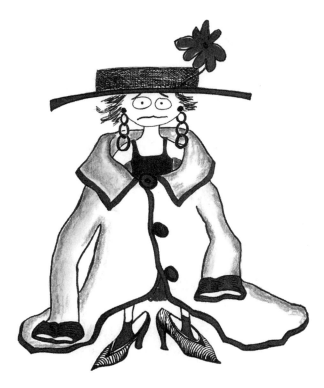

FOR SPITE

There are lots of people you can spite by having sex. Usually they include parents, teachers, ex-girlfriends or ex-boyfriends, or anyone else you think might be upset with your having sex. This is one of the worst reasons to have sex.

FOR BABIES

Having sex is the most efficient way of getting a baby.

FOR FEAR

Boys' and girls' genitals should never be anywhere near each other unless that's what *both* the boy and the girl want. Sometimes a girl wants to say no, but she is afraid. She may be afraid of being left alone. She may be afraid that the boy will physically hurt her if she says no. She may be afraid that he won't believe she cares about him, or that he'll believe she does not find him attractive. She may be afraid to be thought of as childish. She may be afraid he will never ask her out again.

A boy may be afraid he won't be thought of as manly if he doesn't want or insist on sex. He may think that a girl won't like him if he doesn't try.

FOR GIFTS

Your body is not a reward or a present. It is your own gift. But here I am talking about *taking* gifts, or "doing it" for money or presents or favors when you don't really want to. When you do it for money or gifts, you usually don't end up feeling very good about yourself. So, even if someone offers you a trillion quadrillion dollars, remember that nothing would ever be enough.

FOR BOREDOM

A study was once done of what mattered most to teens. Sex was listed eighth, after work, school, friends, and so on. It's often when these other areas of life are difficult that sex becomes an outlet for frustrated energy. It becomes something to fall back on rather than something to move toward. The trouble with sex as a cure for boredom is that if most of your life leaves you feeling down and bored, sex will probably also seem boring. If boredom is what is driving you, it's better to go to a funny movie than to have sex.

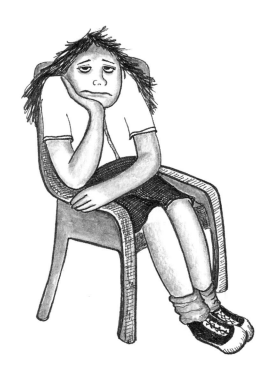

FOR LOVE

As I said in the chapter on love, finding out if what you feel is love is not so easy. Love makes "making love" a different experience from having sex. Love can be a reason to have sex, but it can also be a reason not to. Having sex never "proves" love. Being willing to wait until it is the right time, until both of you are ready, and it is safe, and you both *feel* safe—those may be the "proofs" of love. Love does not change the risks of sexuality. You can still get pregnant, even if you are "doing it for love." And, you can still get AIDS, even if you are "doing it for love."

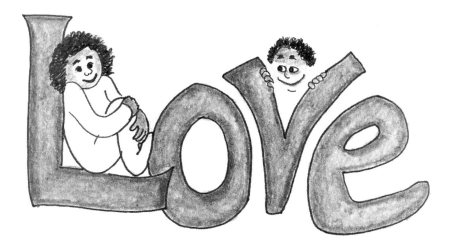

GAY FEELINGS

*T*his is about another kind of sexual experience and, sometimes, another kind of love—that between two boys or two girls. If you ever want to see a lot of adults get uncomfortable, just mention homosexuality.

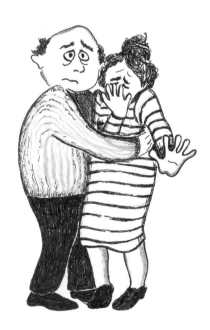

No one really knows why you might be attracted to people of the same sex while others might not. Homosexuality has been a part of most human cultures—and much more accepted at other times and in other places than it sometimes is now. Some people think that homosexuality is something you are born with. Others think it happens as a result of your environment. Still others just see it as one of many choices people make about the expression of their sexuality.

When people talk about homosexuality—or being gay—they are usually talking about two different issues. They mix up *what someone is like* with *who someone likes.* In our culture, we have some pretty rigid ideas of how you should behave if you are male and how you should behave if you are female. We somehow have trouble accepting that if you are a boy, you can be sensitive and gentle, so we just say you aren't being the way boys should be. Well, in reality, a sensitive boy is still very much a boy, and a tough girl is still very much a girl. We never question our "should be's." Then we tease or reject the kids who don't fit into the rigid mold.

Homosexuality is about *who* you are sexually attracted to. It's about girls who prefer to be with girls sexually and boys who prefer to be with boys sexually, and that preference can include the various stages of teen sex. Homosexuality is about boys cuddling with boys, and girls with girls. It's about boys dating boys and girls dating girls. And all the good reasons and bad reasons for you to be with someone apply to homosexual relationships as well as heterosexual relationships (those between a boy and a girl).

Some teens—especially boys—think they have to date to prove they aren't gay. You aren't homosexual just because you don't date. Some boys feel they have to have sex with girls to prove they are not homosexual. Not dating just means you aren't dating, for lots of reasons, and has nothing to do with who you may eventually be with. Dating is just another of our "should be's."

Many people have had some homosexual feelings at some time or other in their lives. (Lots of them won't admit it, though.) In our culture, this is often treated as far worse than wanting to touch yourself or to touch someone of the opposite sex. This is another one of those areas where the anxiety and confusion of adults cause them to react, or overreact, to the thought of a girl with a girl or a boy with a boy. Adults may even flip out about it.

The AIDS epidemic has made some people even more irrational about homosexuality because when the AIDS epidemic was first recognized, the disease seemed to be primarily among male homosexuals. But it was soon discovered that AIDS is also spread by sharing intravenous needles. It is also more and more common among heterosexual men and among women who have sex with infected men.

You don't get AIDS from being a male homosexual. You can get AIDS from any sexual contact with someone—straight or gay, boy or girl—who is infected with the virus, as well as from taking drugs with dirty needles. But for people who were already upset about homosexuality, AIDS became all the more reason to be upset. It's hard to find adults who are relaxed about homosexuality, and so it is not surprising that most teens are uptight about it too.

Sometimes young girls or boys have very close and intimate relationships and care about each other, but do not have a sexual relationship. Other times their relationships do become sexual. As with any relationships, sometimes they last and sometimes they don't. Sometimes boys who want to be with boys continue to prefer men when they grow up—and others grow up to prefer women. And girls who are intimate with other girls either grow up to prefer women or to prefer men. Some like both. These choices or preferences may also change over your lifetime. This can all be *very* confusing to everybody.

It takes a while to get used to having feelings that you might not be expecting. Feelings can sometimes seem so overwhelming that you think you will never feel any other way. As with "going all the way" in heterosexual relationships, people are sexual for all sorts of reasons. So it's a good time to just *do* nothing. The feelings may stay or they may go away. Or they may

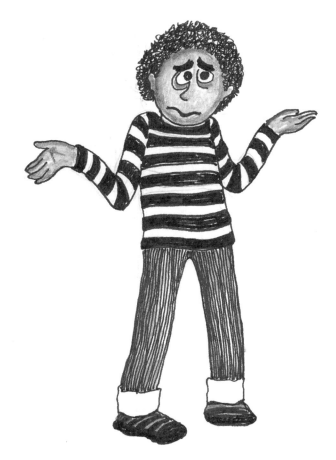

come and go at different times in your life. Give your-self plenty of time to think about how you are feeling, and then decide whether or not you want to act on your feelings.

If you have questions or thoughts about homosexuality, it may be difficult to find others to talk to. Your feelings or thoughts may make you feel isolated and alone. Your thoughts may be very different from those of your family, your friends, or your community. You may be afraid to risk their disapproval by even sharing your thoughts. It is important at least to know that you are not alone in your feelings or questions. As I said earlier, most people have had homosexual thoughts or feelings at some time in their lives, but they are reluctant or unable to talk about them. You may find books to read, or teen helplines to call, or you may be able to find an adult—teacher, doctor, religious counselor—minister, rabbi, priest—whom you can trust. And, as I also said earlier, you have to find *your* answers to how you live your life.

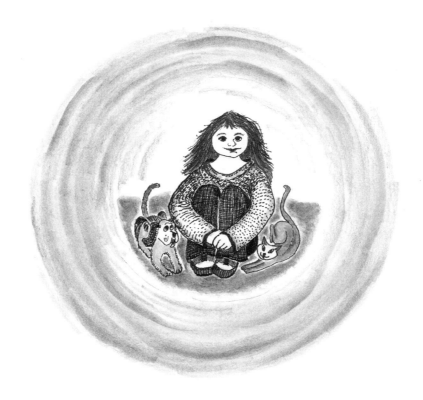

THE PRETEEN'S FIRST BOOK ABOUT LOVE, SEX, AND AIDS

SEX ALL ALONE

*T*ouching yourself . . . masturbation. It's difficult to figure out whether it is considered a worse sin in our society to touch someone else or to touch yourself.

Actually, more people are afraid of touching themselves than of touching someone else. In fact, if they weren't so afraid of touching themselves they might not get into such trouble touching others.

Masturbation is harmless, but not everyone thinks that. Some religions have rules about masturbation. Many adults have strong feelings about it. Most adults—even parents—have at some time touched themselves but are reluctant to admit it. These attitudes make it difficult for you to find someone to talk to if you have questions or worries. Sometimes doctors can be helpful in talking about masturbation. Books for teens often talk about it and can be helpful in answering questions. It can be lonely, having feelings or questions you cannot ask. But you are not alone at all.

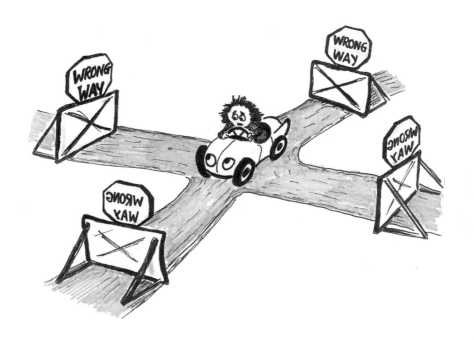

If your shoulder begins to itch, you scratch it. If your wrist begins to ache, you might put a soothing compress or heating pad on it. If your head aches, a parent might suggest aspirin. But, if the itch or ache is in your genitals or private parts (so private even *you* can't look or touch), there's no pill to take and you aren't allowed to make it feel better. *Does this make sense?*

Our attitude toward sex is that if the feelings are "unwanted" or at the wrong time, you have to wish them away, ignore them, or be angry with yourself for having them.

Do your mother and father try to wish away their itches and aches? Usually after adults say, "I wish this headache would go away," they reach for an aspirin.

Just think of all the aspirin bottles in the drug store. Think of all the bottles in your home medicine cabinet. That's because wishing doesn't always work at making discomfort go away. Touching yourself can be a good way to get used to your body—and sexual feelings— without the dangers and confusion of sex play with someone else. Some people actually have more sexual pleasure from masturbating than from having sex.

You can't get diseases from touching yourself; you can't get babies from touching yourself; it causes no harm to you or to anyone else; and it feels good, too.

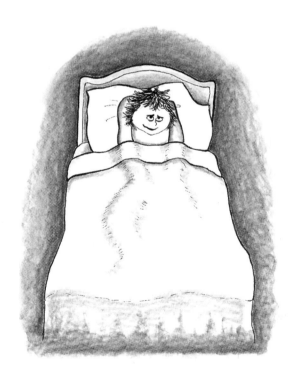

NO SEX

*C*elibacy and *abstinence* are two different terms that refer to not having sex. Celibacy is refraining from any physical or sexual relationship. Abstinence is refraining from having sex in a relationship that may otherwise be physical. The fear of AIDS has led more adults and teens to have relationships that are not sexual at all. Other adults and teens may have physical relationships, but without having sex.

Abstinence is being talked about a lot as one answer to the problems of AIDS (and pregnancy). It recognizes that a teen may feel attracted to another teen and may want to be physical, but may also decide to be safe. Most people—teens and adults—like to feel that they have the option of being sexual with someone else. So, even if they haven't had any sexual experience for weeks, or months, or years, they may still want to think of themselves as being open to some sexual experiences. People may choose celibacy or abstinence because

❀ *THEY AREN'T COMFORTABLE BEING SEXUALLY INTIMATE WITH ANOTHER PERSON.*

❀ *THEY JUST DON'T LIKE SEX OR THE IDEA OF SEX.*

❀ *THEIR MORAL AND RELIGIOUS BELIEFS SUPPORT REFRAINING FROM SEX.*

❀ *THEY ARE AFRAID OF GETTING AIDS.*

❀ *THE RIGHT PERSON HASN'T COME ALONG.*

Being a virgin means you have never had sexual intercourse. We have what we sometimes call a "double standard" for males and females about virginity. Boys are supposed to be very sexual, but girls are not. Boys are often supposed to seek sex without love, while girls are forbidden to have sex without love. This "double standard" leads to some serious problems, like who the boys should be sexual with . . .

For girls, much is often made of whether or not they are virgins, because in most cultures, girls are supposed to be virgins until they marry. However, among many groups of teens, there is pressure on girls *not* to be virgins. A girl's friends may treat her differently, either as if she had passed some test (if she had sex) or as if she is a nerd if she hasn't had sex.

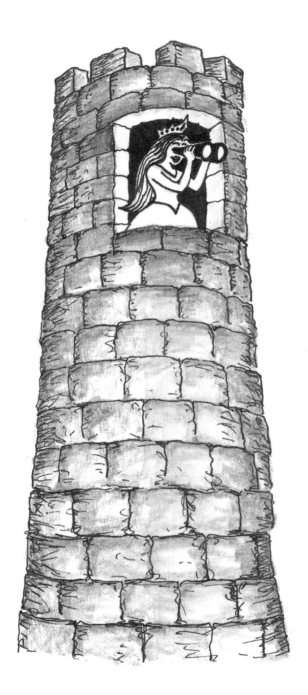

Nothing physically changes in a girl's body after she has intercourse, except for a little tear in the opening of her vagina. However, there is a lot of symbolic meaning in whether she is a virgin. Her feelings about herself may change, depending partly on the circumstances in which she "lost her virginity."

Boys are almost never supposed to be virgins, which is difficult for those boys who just don't want sex at all or just don't feel ready or just haven't met the right girl. Boys (and sometimes even girls) sometimes lie—they pretend that they are not virgins in order to impress friends and to appear to conform.

Someone once said that animals are lucky because they don't know how old they are and therefore they don't have to "act their age." A male horse who is a virgin at 5 years of age doesn't have to "fake it" to his horse friends, and he doesn't have to worry about whether he is "cool."

The point is—there are some very good reasons for girls and boys to postpone having sex. But those reasons are about knowing yourself and others, knowing when and whom to trust, and being able to make the best decision you can. Sometimes you will be happy with your decisions, and sometimes you may behave in ways you later regret. But there really isn't any way to ever know for sure how you will feel tomorrow about what you did or didn't do yesterday.

ABUSES OF SEX

*R*emember the ice cream sundae—the one that would lead to babies if we had been designed differently? Well, ice cream isn't fun if someone is forcing it down your throat. But people can get confused. Girls sometimes think that just because they once ate an ice cream sundae, they are not allowed to refuse it another time. Boys think that because a girl once liked ice cream before, or with someone else, she should like it with them or anyone. The issue isn't ice cream—or sex. The issue is forcing someone to do something with their body, or have something done to their body, that they do not want. Force, either physical or by threat, violates another person's body and dignity and causes him or her great pain. I talked about this before in "Before you even start" (see page 39).

Abuses of sex can lead to a lot of confusion about sexuality. When boys are molested by men or other boys, they sometimes confuse sexual assault with the idea that they are homosexual as a result of the molestation—just like when girls are molested by men or boys, they sometimes confuse the assault with "having sex." When someone forces or pressures you into sex, that's rape. When someone of the opposite sex does it, that's rape. When someone of the same sex does it, that's rape. It's not homosexuality. Rape is rape, whatever sex you are, or whatever the sex of the person who pressures or forces you into sex you do not want.

An activity can be either pleasurable or terrifying, depending on whether you are in control of what is being done to you. For instance,

⇨ *SWIMMING UNDER WATER CAN BE LOTS OF FUN. BEING THROWN IN THE WATER AND HELD UNDER IS TERRIFYING.*

⇨ *RIDING IN AN ELEVATOR CAN BE FUN. BEING LOCKED IN ONE MAY BE TERRIFYING.*

⇨ *SKYDIVING CAN BE FUN. BEING PUSHED OUT OF AN AIRPLANE IS TERRIFYING.*

Because sex when you are feeling loving or intimate or sexual can be fun, some people think it should be fun anytime. But, like kissing, or swimming under water, or riding in elevators, or parachuting out of airplanes, when you have no control, it is no fun at all.

Sometimes there seems to be a fine line between *play* and *abuse.* You can think it is play, but the other person can feel it is abuse. Or you can start out with what seems like play and it can get out of hand. So, whenever you need to say "no" or whenever someone says "no" to you, that is the time to stop. You can hurt someone without meaning to. You can get hurt without someone meaning to hurt you. Most abuse between teens happens when you don't stop when the other person tells you to stop.

Words can also be abusive. Using profanity or "dirty" language *at* someone can be abusive, even if it isn't meant to be. When the person using the language is in a position of authority over a teen, or child, then it is always abuse. It is abuse whether the person is a teacher, doctor, coach, parent, bus driver, older teen, or boss.

Sexual abuse affects you for a very long time, sometimes for the rest of your life. If you have been abused, you may have some of these problems:

✪ Trouble sleeping, sometimes with nightmares.
✪ Fears of being alone, at home, in elevators, in a room.
✪ Fear of the dark.
✪ Fear of any reminders of the time or place where you were abused. For instance, if you were abused in a park you may be afraid of parks, even when other people are around and you know you are safe. If you were abused on a holiday (for

instance, on the Fourth of July) you may have fears every Fourth of July. In other words, reminders of the abuse bring on the painful feelings from the time of the abuse.

✪ Trouble relaxing. You may startle easily and not know why. When someone walks up to you from behind you may suddenly jump, even when there is no reason to be afraid.

✪ Trouble with any sexual feelings. This was also talked about earlier in the book in "Before you even start" (page 39).

✪ Feeling depressed and like you have no future.

✪ Trying to fight the fears of sexuality by being reckless about sex.

✪ Feeling confused about your sexuality, especially if the abuser is of the same sex.

✪ Feeling worthless.

It may be hard to understand why sexual abuse has such terrible and long-lasting effects on boys and girls, men and women. But, whether or not we understand why, the effects are there. Sexual violation is not like any other abuse. The crossing of sexual boundaries between people, whether in word or touch, seems to cause deeper wounds and greater shame than any other kinds of abuse. *The person who commits the crime of sexual abuse seems to pass on the shame and humiliation to the victim.* It makes no sense, but it seems to

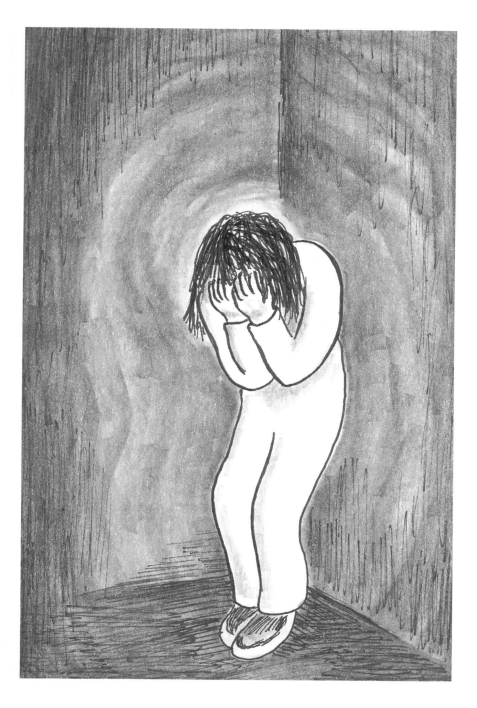

be that way. In other words, the victim often ends up feeling guilty, even though she or he has done nothing to deserve either the abuse or the shame.

Abuse feelings don't go away with time. In fact, they usually get worse. Fears get worse, the effects on sexuality get worse, and feelings of worthlessness get worse. Sometimes people lose the memory of abuse, only to have it reappear years later.

Secrets grow well in the dark. The thought of light—of telling someone what happened—becomes more frightening. You become more isolated, believing you are the only one with these feelings.

Abuse is common, unfortunately, and therefore its effects are common. Among any group of teens, more than one has probably been abused.

Many people are prepared to help you with problems of abuse these days. Abuse is being talked about more. Adults have become more aware of what happens to kids, and what happened to them when they were kids. Abuse has to be talked about, sometimes with other teens, with adults, and with family or doctors. Especially because the effects last so long, it is important that you get help as soon as possible so you can go about enjoying the rest of your life.

SEX AND AIDS

*Y*ou've all heard of AIDS! Even if you've had a bag over your head, the message has probably gotten through that the *human immunodeficiency virus* (HIV) causes an incurable disease called *acquired immunodeficiency syndrome* (AIDS). The virus that causes AIDS travels from the inside of one person's body to the inside of another person's body. It doesn't live in air, on toilet seats, or on the surface of your skin. It's home is in body fluids: blood, semen (the fluid in a male that carries sperm—as well as other little organisms like viruses), and saliva (spit). And, when it goes from one person into another, it causes an infection. It has to go *into* your body or through openings in your skin and then into your bloodstream for you to get AIDS. The main ways in which preteens and teens get AIDS are by having sex or by sharing needles to do drugs. In both of those situations, HIV travels from the inside of one body to the inside of another. If a woman is pregnant, the virus

79

can also infect the baby before it is born. In fact, the virus can cause AIDS in the baby long before the woman herself knows she has the virus.

How does AIDS kill you? The virus attacks the cells that usually protect you from getting sick. These are called *T cells,* because they are related to the thymus gland (a gland that helps the body's immune system). The T cells are responsible for recognizing and destroying harmful agents that come into the body. But when the T cells are destroyed, the body is open to many other illnesses. If you have AIDS, ordinary illnesses like a cold can kill you.

Pretend your body is a fort with strong high walls. Patrolling the fort are hundreds of thousands of soldiers—the T cells. These soldiers are on the lookout for foreign invaders who are trying to take over the fort. Constantly surrounding the fort are small groups of these potential invaders, looking for a chance to sneak past the guards.

Now pretend that a terrible sickness has affected the guards. They lose their vision and their voices so they cannot even warn others that there are enemies closing in (the T cells lose their ability to warn other cells). They lose their weapons (T cells are unable to destroy invading organisms). The foreign invaders overwhelm the guards and the fort is taken—except in this case, the disease is AIDS and the fort is *you.* It's HIV that causes the terrible sickness of the T cell guards. HIV can also lie in wait for many years before it affects the T cells. You can be infected for 10 years without having the sickness, just waiting.

AIDS comes from a *virus,* but you get the virus from a *person.* The risks of AIDS are very great, but "being careful" isn't always easy, or enough. It's tough to be with someone you care about—enough to want to kiss—and have to act as though that person has AIDS.

The problem is even more complicated because, as I said before, the AIDS-causing virus may live quietly in your body for 10 years or longer without your being aware of it, and without your being sick. So, being healthy, *feeling* healthy, doesn't mean you are not infected. And someone else can look and be healthy but still carry the virus—and infect you—without their being aware of being infected or contagious.

A blood test is used to tell whether someone is carrying the AIDS virus. But even that is not so simple, because the blood test doesn't always show the infection right away. In other words, you have to be infected for a while, maybe up to 6 months, before the virus will show up in the test. That means that someone can have a blood test for the AIDS virus and the test can be negative, but the person can still be carrying the virus. You can get the virus and even pass it on to someone else before your blood test is positive or before you even get sick from the virus.

Whether we assume that everyone else *has* AIDS or

that everyone *could* have AIDS, there are three basic questions which need answering:

❀ *WHAT DO I NEED TO KNOW ABOUT MYSELF?*

❀ *WHAT DO I NEED TO KNOW ABOUT THE OTHER PERSON?*

❀ *WHAT DO I NEED TO KNOW ABOUT THE VIRUS?*

WHAT DO I NEED TO KNOW ABOUT MYSELF?

Remember the car, the one you only get one of in a lifetime? Remember risk taking and thinking you are immortal? They are part of what you have to know about yourself. You need to ask yourself about your own risk taking:

▷ *DO I TEND TO TAKE RISKS?*

▷ *DO I TAKE RISKS THINKING THAT NOTHING COULD HAPPEN TO ME?*

▷ *DO I CARE WHAT HAPPENS TO ME? DO I THINK IT IS O.K. TO CARE WHAT HAPPENS TO ME?*

▷ *AM I AFRAID TO HAVE SOMEONE ELSE KNOW THAT I CARE ABOUT WHAT HAPPENS TO ME?*

▷ *AM I AFRAID NOT TO DO WHAT OTHERS WANT?*

If you're having trouble thinking about your own safety, think about your best friend, or think about your little sister or brother and what you think about that person's being safe. Sometimes it's easier to worry about the safety of others than about ourselves. For instance, teens who smoke cigarettes might be horrified to see their younger brothers or sisters smoking.

AIDS is about risks. AIDS is about whether you feel it is O.K. to take care of yourself. Think about what advice you would give your best friend, or little brother or sister, and then take the advice yourself!

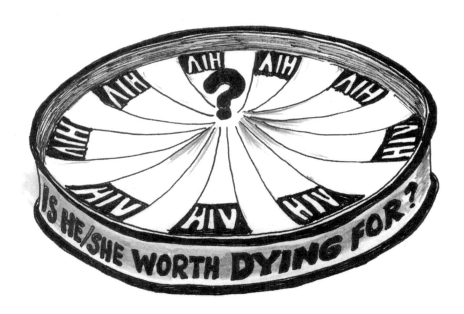

WHAT DO I NEED TO KNOW ABOUT THE OTHER PERSON?

This is both tough and easy, because basically you only need to know if the other person carries HIV. But finding that out is not so easy, because no one wants to talk about it. It's also hard because you can carry the AIDS virus for many years without being sick, and therefore without knowing you are infected. And, you can even carry the AIDS-causing virus for a while before the lab test will show its presence.

How do you even ask about AIDS? How do you know if the other person is telling the truth? This may be one of the toughest challenges for any teen, or adult for that matter—asking someone else about AIDS. Because the disease is associated with sex, drugs, and homosexuality, it may seem like an insult to ask someone about AIDS. And yet—in spite of its making good sense to ask, some people might be offended at your asking—even though they shouldn't be—and even though they might have the same worries. So then you are left wondering whether it is better to risk offending someone else or to risk getting AIDS. . . . If the other person is really that close to you, close enough so you are thinking about being sexual with each other, that person shouldn't put you in the position of making that choice. Can you really imagine someone you care about saying, "I'd like to have sex, but let's not talk about AIDS!"

Now that's nuts!

Remember the bag over David's head? Well, sometimes we all act like David in relation to AIDS. We pretend there is no problem.

Now, who is this person you are thinking about being sexual with? Is this a friend? Friends don't put you in danger, and they don't even make you have to sweat asking about AIDS. If this person is not a friend—why are you even thinking about letting fluids from inside his or her body get inside yours? Remember how you get AIDS? Insides to insides—blood to blood, spit to spit, semen to vagina—in lots of places.

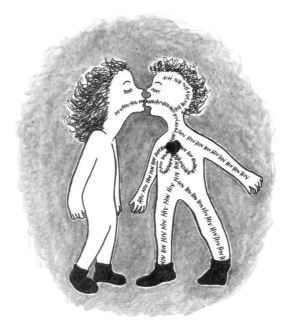

But also remember that someone can be infected and not even know it.

The question of whether someone is telling the truth—well, that has to do with how well you know each other. People who lie usually lie to lots of people. People who are generally truthful are probably truthful to you too. It's probably not realistic to get a lie detector test to see if someone is lying about AIDS. But, if you think you might want someone to take a lie detector test it's probably because you think the person might not be telling the truth. And if you think that—step back and be cautious, very cautious! Wishing for a lie detector test should be a warning that trust is very, very low. You have a right to protect yourself!

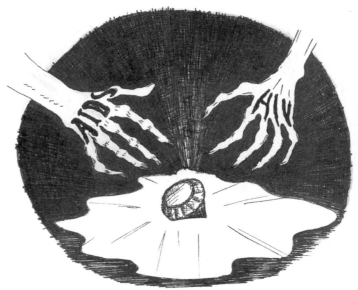

Love doesn't protect you from AIDS either. You can be in love—the ice cube can indeed have a diamond inside—but you can still get AIDS.

WHAT DO I NEED TO KNOW ABOUT THE VIRUS?

As I said before, HIV—the virus that causes AIDS—lives in body fluids. So knowing about the virus is knowing about fluids. Viruses aren't really like fish, but in the same way that fish die outside water, the virus dies outside body fluids. If you want to catch a fish you have to go where there is water. If you want to find the AIDS-causing virus, you have to go where there are body fluids. The virus has to have a way of getting from one body to another, through the fluids. It can't dry out or it will die, like a fish out of water. It also has to have a way *into* your body in order for the virus to infect you. That's why just hanging out with someone who has AIDS or touching the skin of someone who has AIDS doesn't spread the infection. You can get colds from being in a room with someone with a cold. That's because the cold viruses live in the *air*. So, if you breathe air with the cold virus, you may get a cold. But the AIDS virus doesn't live in the air, or on your skin—only in body fluids: blood, semen, and saliva.

Remember—fluids to fluids, insides to insides.

HOW THE AIDS VIRUS CAN SPREAD

What are the major ways the virus that causes AIDS gets into your body?

KISSING

Kissing can spread AIDS if you have any sores at all, even tiny ones in your mouth, or if you have chapped lips, or bite your lip, or chew your gums. In other words, there has to be a way for the virus to get *inside* your body, into your bloodstream. In kissing, the virus from someone with AIDS travels with their saliva into your mouth. If you have any tiny sores or chapped lips or burns, then the virus goes through those openings and into your bloodstream. And then you know the rest.

SEXUAL INTERCOURSE

Sexual intercourse is *the* major way that the virus travels between people. The virus goes from the semen into the other person's body. When semen goes into a girl's vagina, the virus can travel through any tiny tears or cuts or rubs in the lining of her vagina and on into the bloodstream—where HIV goes on eventually to kill the T cells. The same thing can happen if semen ends up in the mouth. When boys have sex with each other, the semen can end up in the mouth or in the anus (the butt) and also go through tiny openings. Then the virus goes into the bloodstream and on to kill off the T cells.

NEEDLES

Needles spread AIDS when they are shared while people are taking drugs. HIV likes blood. It grows well and travels well in blood. So, if you take a needle that someone else has used to inject drugs and put it into your body, the virus travels from the dirty needle into your bloodstream, and eventually kills off the T cells. This is also why blood transfusions, if the blood is not free of the virus, can also cause AIDS.

So, the major way of avoiding AIDS is to avoid body fluids from someone else. If you don't kiss or have sex or take drugs—or have blood transfusions—you don't get AIDS.

If you **are** *going to be sexual, then at least there are ways to reduce the risk of AIDS.*

SAFE SEX

Safe sex is the term used to describe ways to decrease the risk of AIDS while still being sexual with someone who has or who might have AIDS. Safe sex means setting up a barrier between any openings into your body and the other person's fluids. Safe sex is about trying to prevent the spread of the virus from one person to the next:

✪ Don't exchange saliva in kissing. . . . A dry kiss on the cheek seems to be relatively safe.
✪ Use condoms for any sexual activity involving semen. As long as the semen stays in the condom (be careful not to spill it and that the condom

doesn't break), the virus can't get into another person's body. Some condoms have been found to have defects—little holes—that let semen through, so you can't always trust condoms to protect you.

✪ If you are having sex over any other surfaces or holes in the body, use a plastic barrier, like a dental shield (something like heavy plastic wrap), so semen and saliva can't enter the body.

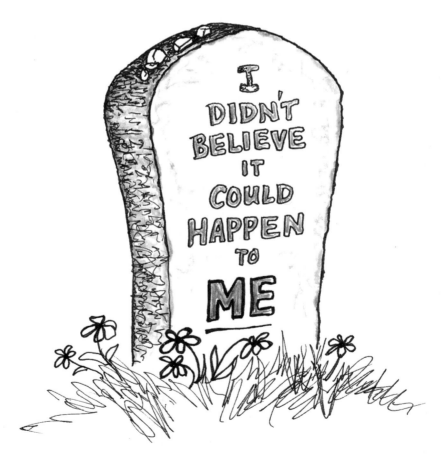

It may seem like all of this would spoil the "fun" and "spontaneity" of sexual activity, but it's not as bad as losing T cells, getting AIDS, having no fun at all—and maybe even dying. Remember, back at the beginning of this book when I asked, "Why take care of your body?" It's still the only one you've got—and the only one you'll ever get. So, we all have to either take care of our bodies, or risk losing them . . .

THE END AND THE BEGINNING

*R*emember the path at the beginning of this book—the path through the fun, fear, and confusion of sexuality? Well, for each person—grown-up, teen, or preteen—the path is similar and also different. But this path is about your own thoughts, values, dreams, wishes, feelings, fears, beliefs, religion, and experiences. It is about *you*. There are choices about sexuality that are within your control to make, as well as events that happen to you that are beyond your control. But what you do with them, where you take yourself, depends on *you* and who the people are who join you on your path.

There are road signs for all of us as we live our lives, signs that should not be ignored because they really can guide us through the good times and bad, the happy times and lonely times. Don't ignore the road signs:

- ♥ *BELIEVE IN YOURSELF.*

- ♥ *ASK FOR HELP WHEN YOU FEEL LOST.*

- ♥ *SLOW DOWN WHEN THINGS ARE MOVING TOO FAST.*

- ♥ *LOOK FOR FRIENDS YOU CAN TRUST TO BE WITH YOU ON THE PATH.*

- ♥ *PROTECT YOURSELF FROM DANGER.*

- ♥ *STOP WHEN YOU WANT TO STOP.*

- ♥ *DON'T GIVE UP YOUR OWN PATH FOR SOMEONE ELSE'S.*

- ♥ *DON'T BE AFRAID TO BE ALONE.*

- ♥ *TRUST IN YOUR ABILITY TO MAKE CHOICES.*

As for sex and safety, if you have sex, you want to minimize the risks. You do this by decisions as to who you are with, what you decide to do, and then how to be safe about any sexual activity. Those decisions are equally important in risks to your body, such as AIDS, and in emotional risks. There is great happiness to be had in relationships, especially ones of love, but there are always risks too—risks of physical dangers like AIDS (which can kill you) and risks of great emotional pain. For all risks, physical and emotional, the answers are to know your partner and to also be careful.

We all live in a constant tug-of-war that goes on inside. Pulling in one direction are all our feelings, sensations, and wishes for pleasure. Pulling in the other direction are fears, caution, and the voices we hear telling us what we think our parents or teachers would be telling us. Caught in the middle, we try to balance the two sides of ourselves. If the "feelings" let go, so that caution takes over completely, then we can be without fun and pleasure. If the caution lets go and feelings take over completely, then we run great risks of danger to body and emotion. Either way we fall flat on our faces, so we just have to stay in the tug-of-war and keep struggling for some balance. Either way, you are still walking a tightrope.

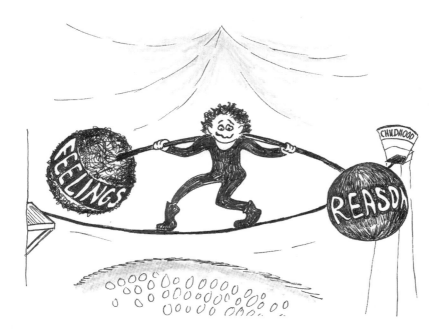

If you are reading this book, or thinking about sex, you are facing a great adventure. While every one of us copes with questions of sexuality, in the end, we each also have to find our own answers. How we live our sexual lives is not so different from how we live the rest of our lives. The search for answers, for what it all means, may be as rich as the answers themselves. In the meantime, and while you are on your quest, I offer some advice:

⇨ *TAKE GOOD CARE OF YOUR CAR.*

⇨ *WATCH OUT FOR THOSE ICE CREAM SUNDAES.*

⇨ *DON'T HAVE A BABY UNLESS YOU WANT TO.*

⇨ *AVOID PUTTING PAPER BAGS OVER YOUR HEAD.*

⇨ *DON'T JUMP OUT OF AIRPLANES UNLESS YOU REALLY WANT TO.*

⇨ *DON'T HOLD OTHER PEOPLE UNDER WATER.*

⇨ *GUARD YOUR T CELLS.*

⇨ *IF YOU DON'T KNOW WHAT TO DO, WAIT TILL THE ICE CUBE MELTS. IT'S O.K. TO LOOK FOR THE DIAMONDS.*

⇨ *YOU ARE A GIFT.*

And finally:

⇨ *DON'T BE TOO HARD ON YOUR PARENTS. THEY ARE STILL RE-COVERING FROM BEING TEENS THEMSELVES.*

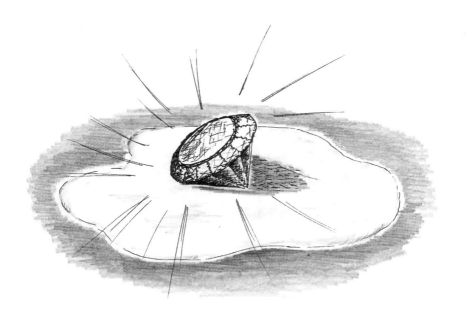